Fifteen Secrets to Becoming a Successful Chiropractor

ISBN 1-58961-360-0

Published by PageFree Publishing, Inc.
www.pagefreepublishing.com
109 South Farmer Street
Otsego, MI 49078

Fifteen Secrets to Becoming a Successful Chiropractor

Dr. John L. Reizer

Dedication

This book is dedicated to my late friend and mentor, Dr. Vincent Toma.

Table of Contents

About The Author

Dr. John Reizer is a 1986 magna cum laude graduate of Sherman College of Straight Chiropractic. Born in Lakewood, New Jersey in 1963, he returned home to his native state after graduating from college and opened two successful chiropractic offices. Dr. Reizer returned to Sherman College as a member of the teaching faculty in 1998 after twelve years of private practice. He is currently an Assistant Professor of Clinical Sciences at Sherman College and practices in the college's health center supervising interns who are preparing to enter the field of chiropractic.

Other books by Dr. John Reizer:

Up and Running – Opening a Chiropractic Office
ISBN 1-93025-270-6

_Chiropractic Made Simple – Working With the Controlling Laws
of Nature_
ISBN 1-58961-039-3

Disclaimer

The author and the publisher would like to acknowledge that this book represents only the views of the author. At no time whatsoever does the author claim to be a spokesperson for any chiropractic college, chiropractic organization, or for individual chiropractors. The opinions expressed in this book are a product of the author's own experience as a practicing doctor of chiropractic and instructor.

Introduction

My name is Dr. John Reizer and I have been a chiropractor since 1986. I have experienced what some people would consider a significant amount of professional success while wearing many different hats throughout my chiropractic career. I have been a student, a private practitioner, a college instructor, a lecturer, an author, and a practice consultant to other doctors. Although many of the professional accomplishments I have been able to attain over the years have been a direct result of genuine opportunities which have crossed my path, I wouldn't say that all of these accomplishments just magically materialized for me. I have been very fortunate in that I have been able to capitalize on certain opportunities that have presented themselves at different times in my life. Not all of these situations however, have turned out to be wonderful success stories for me. In fact some of these so-called opportunities that I acted upon have caused me significant financial and emotional distress. For the most part, however, I have been blessed with positive outcomes when making extremely important life decisions.

Throughout my career I have met many successful chiropractors. These individuals have taught me invaluable lessons about what it means to be successful in both professional and personal life settings. One very important observation I was able to make from my various dealings with these highly successful practitioners was that they all shared common personality traits that ultimately led to their successful ways. Obviously some of these men and women were more successful than others. Some of them were also successful in different ways from one another. Success is a unique word and very often people will have a different understanding of what it means to be successful.

Quite a few people in our society define success solely by the amount of wealth an individual has amassed in his or her lifetime. Americans, for the most part, have a materialistic mentality and so it is easy to understand why so many people in our own country believe that in order to be successful an individual has to have large reserves of money in the bank. If this theory of success was actually true in every instance it would be very easy to pick out all of the successful people in the world.

Although financial independence seems like a wonderful situation to experience it is by no means the final verdict on how successful an individual is in a particular arena. I think most of us would agree that there are many successful people in the world who happen to be affluent. But on the other side of the fence, there are also many folks out there who consider themselves very successful and are simultaneously suffering from a shortage of currency in their personal bank accounts. Keep in mind that how we perceive success or a lack of success is largely dependent on our definition of the word.

For me, the definition of success is quite simple to understand. I believe that people can be considered successful whenever they are able to achieve personal goals which they previously set out to accomplish. Sometimes these goals are major milestones in their lives and sometimes they are much smaller goals that are mere stepping stones to bigger and better things to come in the future. The size or capacity of the goal is really not that important. Success can be measured in every human being and it is based on a person's ability to accomplish his or her own agenda within his or her own personal timetable. In my opinion the word failure describes just another opportunity to try something over again so that you can ultimately become successful at attaining the objective at a later date. The only people in the world who are not successful are those individuals who give up on becoming successful.

Throughout the many years that I have been involved with this profession I have been trying to analyze the various components that make chiropractors successful. It should be noted that I have had the unique opportunity to view many practitioners as well as future practitioners in an academic setting. I am now able to predict with a high degree of accuracy which students will become successful in practice. I can also predict which students will struggle as chiropractic practitioners. You might wonder if I am clairvoyant or a psychic. I am neither. But I do know the signs to look for. I know the *Fifteen Secrets to Becoming a Successful Chiropractor.*

I understand that many people reading this introduction may be skeptical regarding my claim to be able to predict the probable level of success a particular doctor will achieve. This, in reality, is not that difficult to do and after reading the information in this book, you, the reader, will be able to do the same. More importantly you will be able to develop a mindset that will help you to achieve a much higher degree of success within your personal life as well as your professional practice. I have discovered a secret formula for success which I have used time and time again in many areas of my life. It always works and if you can follow the very simple advice that I write here, you will always be successful in whatever you set out to do.

I have broken this formula down into fifteen individual chapters and it will help tremendously if you read each chapter in the chronological order in which it appears in the text. Please do not jump around through the various chapters. In this way you will get the maximum results and will understand more clearly what will be expected of you in order to become the very successful chiropractor you deserve to be.

-Dr. John Reizer

#1

Create Realistic Personal Goals

1

Create Realistic Personal Goals

The first secret to becoming a successful chiropractor is quite simply being able to visualize yourself in such a capacity. Perhaps one of the best ways to accomplish such a feat is by creating a set of personal goals. Setting personal goals and making them realistic enough so that you can eventually attain them in a reasonable amount of time will help to facilitate the process of achieving your own personal and professional success.

There is a definite methodology to consider when setting goals. It is not something that should be rushed into blindly without careful planning. If you are serious about being successful in a particular area of your life you will need to take the time to carefully think about what exactly it is that you want to accomplish.

Visualization techniques are extremely useful when creating goals. If you cannot visualize the objective you are trying to accomplish, it is rather unlikely that you will be able to succeed in your venture. Once you are able to visualize where you would like to go or what you would like to accomplish, you will need to take a mental snapshot of that image. It is important that you capture, in your mind's eye, the essence of that mental image and that you never forget it.

Next, you will need to write down, on a piece of paper, the types of personal goals you would like to accomplish. You should begin by writing a rough draft of your goals into a simple paragraph. Writing the information down on paper helps to make the intangible tangible. This is a crucial step in the goal-setting process because it takes the visual picture which you created and transforms it directly into your total perceived reality.

When writing your personal goals, it is important to remember that they should be constructed realistically. You should also avoid making them too large. Really big goals should be reduced to smaller objectives. This will prevent you from becoming overwhelmed by the size of a particular task. Keep in mind that large or small unrealistic goals can lead a person into a corner filled with frustration which will ultimately prevent the individual from becoming successful in accomplishing his or her objectives.

Keep your goals very specific. You do not want to write down a bunch of objectives that are too general or vague. This can lead to problems later on. It is also important to make the goals very private and applicable to only one person – you! Do not, under any circumstances, allow friends or family members to help you author these objectives. You are the person who has taken the mental snapshot of where you want to be and therefore you should be the person writing down the pertinent information.

I believe it is extremely important to construct schedules for your goals along with specific dates that you expect to attain them. Goals that are set without immediate timetables are difficult to achieve. By attaching schedules to your goals, you can pace yourself and are able to track the level of your progress over time. A schedule also allows you the flexibility to modify a specific goal should this become necessary.

The next step in this process is to prioritize your goals. This will help you classify and then separate your primary objectives from the far less important objectives. This can also be a big help in keeping you focused on the bigger picture while simultaneously allowing you to remain realistic in your approach so that you can take care of business that needs to be dealt with.

Now that you have your *preliminary goals* prioritized into clear, specific, personalized objectives, you might want to assess whether or not any modifications need to be made at this point. Do your written goals represent the visual image that you previously constructed? If the written and the visual components are a match, you are in good shape. If the written and visual components are not congruent you will definitely need to modify the written information so that it matches the visual snapshot in your mind. You will need to take the *preliminary goals* and adjust them accordingly. In either scenario the written and visual components must mirror one another. Once this is achieved the *preliminary goals* are then referred to as the *adjusted goals*.

When your *adjusted goals* have been finalized you will want to identify any barriers or possible obstacles that might prevent you from accomplishing what you have placed on paper. Obstacles are simply the non-important items in our lives that some people choose to focus on when they take their eyes off the major goal they are trying to attain. These obstacles are mental illusions that human beings often construct for various reasons. Examples of such obstacles are laziness, procrastination, as well as a multitude of other excuses that work their way into the equation. I believe that in many instances, people will construct such barriers because they are afraid of being successful. Once individuals become cognizant of these barriers which prevent them from achieving their personal goals, they are often able to become more productive. They are then able to reposition their line of vision back in the direction of the original objective and the obstacles suddenly and miraculously vanish.

You have now created a written blue print which will help to ensure your future success. It is going to be imperative that you stay loyal to your cause. It is one thing to write down a game plan and quite another thing to execute the plan to a level that is necessary to win the game.

It will be important for you to periodically track the level of your progress, as well as to review the goals you have written down. You should also continue to try and visualize the results you are trying to achieve on a regular basis. Remember that this is only the first secret in the formula and that we have much more territory to cover.

I have prepared worksheets on the next few pages of this book to help you with the process of setting up your written goals. I would suggest making several copies of the worksheets so that you can work with a large number of goals at the same time. After you complete the worksheets, you will be asked to construct a graph which will help you to track your progress. The use of a graph (a visual tool) will be helpful in keeping you focused and excited about accomplishing the various personal objectives you are working toward. Measuring your progress along with repetitiously reviewing your goals on a daily basis will allow you to form positive habits that will greatly increase your chances of being successful in completing your prioritized objectives.

Written Goals Worksheet

1. Write down in a simple paragraph the goals that you have previously visualized.

2. Each major goal should then be broken down into smaller goals or objectives.

    a)

    b)

    c)

3. Create a schedule and an estimated date of completion for each of the smaller goals that you listed.

    a)

    b)

    c)

4. Prioritize the smaller goals that you have listed.

    1)

    2)

    3)

5. Do the preliminary, prioritized, smaller goals match or represent the visual image you have made in your mind?

Yes ( )   No ( )

6. If the answer to question number five is "YES" you will proceed to item number eight on this worksheet. If the answer to item number five is "NO" you will need to adjust your preliminary goals in the spaces provided in item number seven.

7. Rewrite your smaller goals so that they are congruent with the visual image you constructed prior to writing the original paragraph on this worksheet.

1)

2)

3)

8. List your finalized "Adjusted Goals" which match your mental snapshot.

1)

2)

3)

9. List possible barriers/obstacles that might prevent you from reaching your "Adjusted Goals."

Homework Assignment

Construct a chart that displays your final "Adjusted Goals" in a prioritized order. Position each of the "Adjusted Goals" on the left side of the chart. You might also want to indicate in (parenthesis) a few of the obstacles that you have identified which correspond to each "Adjusted Goal." Listing the obstacles on the chart will help you to remain focused and aware of possible problems that might show up later on down the road. On the bottom of the chart, make a time line or calendar which represents the schedule you have laid out in order for the "Adjusted Goals" to be completed. When you proceed from left to right on the bottom portion of the chart this will represent the days or months that are passing. On the right side of the chart you will make a column which will represent your current level of success in reaching the "Adjusted Goals." This column should be designed so that the higher up the page you are positioned the closer you will be to attaining your various goals.

After your chart is completed, you should be able to see for each goal a linear representation of your progress over time. Use different colored pencils or markers for each goal in order that you can track multiple objectives at the same time.

A sample chart has been prepared on the next page for your convenience. Please refer to this example when designing your own model. It is also advisable to place your chart in a location where you can view it on a regular basis.

SAMPLE CHART

Success

Personal Goals   **Try Again**

Time Allocated

2

Write a Mission Statement

2

Write a Mission Statement

The second secret to becoming a successful chiropractor is learning how to write a clear and concise mission statement for your professional practice. A mission statement is a very brief explanation to your patients and staff about the objectives your company is trying to achieve.

There are many businesses functioning within the United States that have not taken the time to create a proper mission statement. These businesses are operating without a clear understanding of what it is they are trying to accomplish for their clients.

I like to think of a mission statement as a group of goals that are similar to the objectives that we set in our personal lives. In actuality the mission statement is very often an extension of the personal goals that we do set. There is however a subtle difference between the two sets of objectives. The difference between the two is simply that personal goals are objectives that an individual is trying to attain while obviously the objectives contained and described within the mission statement document are goals that a particular company is trying to achieve for their clients.

Items to Consider

There are a number of items that you should consider before ever picking up a pen to begin writing this document. The first order of business which will be paramount to the success of preparing the mission statement will be to have a clear understanding of the service you will be performing for your patients. Within the chiropractic profession, there are various practice objectives that have managed to get lumped together. To a layperson, our profession might seem much more unified than it actually is. A common misconception within the lay community is that all chiropractic practitioners regularly offer identical services. Those of us who are residents within the house of chiropractic know a much different story. We realize that there are many practitioners within the profession who have very different practice objectives from one another. Because you are going to be a service-oriented company you must have a great understanding of the service you will be performing. You must be very specific in describing this service to patients and members of your staff so that there is no room for misunderstanding or confusion about the company objectives. It would also be a good idea to explain within the mission statement how your company's service is different from other health related professions.

Remember to always keep things simple and try to choose a writing style that reflects your thoughts and ideas clearly. I would highly recommend that you take the time to view numerous mission statements from a wide assortment of well-established companies. Also take the time to observe the various components which make up these documents. Look at how the sentences have been constructed. In most instances, if the statements have been prepared properly, you will discover that these writings are all similar in that they have been authored to allow the company objectives to be explained in just a few short sentences. Brevity can certainly be a wonderful thing. By being brief and to the point your patients will instantly understand what information you are trying to pass on to them.

Advice from Others

Constructive input from knowledgeable colleagues, staff members, as well as from other individuals who possess business organizational skills can be helpful to your cause. Although it is not a good idea to have outsiders help you when you are writing your personal goals, the same cannot be said when it comes to designing the mission statement. Very often brainstorming sessions by your staff members and associate doctors can provide tremendous productivity, creativity, and a finished document with which everyone in the company is much more likely to resonate. When members of a company or your office staff directly contribute to the creation of the mission statement there is a good chance that all of these people are going to feel very positive about the objectives being promoted within the company. This is a wonderful opportunity to create peace and harmony within the office setting.

A Sample Statement

Each college semester I teach a *Chiropractic Philosophical Applications* course which I happen to enjoy very much. I often require students in that course to write their own theoretical mission statements. In direct opposition to the advice which I offer in this chapter, I have my students write their statements on the spur of the moment without any prior warning. The reason I do this is twofold. The first reason is because I want to drive home the point that a mission statement is not an easy document to write. The second reason is because I want students to begin thinking about setting professional practice objectives while they are still in school. After we conclude the exercise, I then give the students a homework assignment which requires them to take the necessary time to prepare a proper document. If you want to be a successful chiropractor you need to start thinking and acting like a successful chiropractor. This includes being able to identify your professional mission as well as being able to teach it to everyone who enters your place of business.

Below is a version of a mission statement that I have used in my own private practice for many years. I hope that this will be helpful to you when you begin to write your own statement. Keep in mind that the philosophical objectives which I subscribe to are of my own preference. It is not important that you adhere to my philosophical rationale. It is however, very important that you adhere to some form of rationale and that you incorporate such a rationale into your own practice objectives.

Mission Statement

The Reizer Chiropractic Center has a unique healthcare mission which specializes in the location, analysis, and correction of vertebral subluxations. Vertebral subluxations occur when the spinal bones become slightly misaligned from one another and place pressure on adjacent spinal nerves. Vertebral subluxations are detrimental to the optimal functioning of the nervous system and they are also an inhibiting factor in the full expression of health in all human beings.

The examination procedures and corrective techniques utilized by Dr. Reizer are all instrumental in achieving the professional mission of this office which is to correct these harmful conditions in our patients' spines. Dr. Reizer does not offer to diagnose diseases or medical conditions in patients as this objective is outside the scope of chiropractic.

This is a very concise explanation of my professional practice objectives. In two short paragraphs I have communicated to the reader what I do in my office and more importantly the reason why I am doing it. I have also explained what I do not do and how my objectives are different from other health-related fields.

It is my suggestion that you place your mission statement in a very conspicuous location within your place of business. I would hang it on a wall in the office waiting room or perhaps in the room where you perform your patient consultations. It should definitely be in an area that patients and staff members frequent. I would also take the time to produce a high quality copy of the mission statement and have it professionally framed.

It is also a very good idea to have copies of your mission statement printed within some of your office brochures and other related literature that you give out to patients. I would also read the mission statement to new patients and repeat it once again when doing group health talks.

3

Become an Effective Communicator

3

Become an Effective Communicator

The third secret to becoming a successful chiropractor is learning how to master the art of communication. Being an effective communicator will help you to create a non-stressful environment within your practice.

Many doctors have difficulty expressing themselves to other professionals and their patients. The free exchange of various ideas between individuals is essential to the overall success of personal and professional relationships. Since relationships are essential to the success of any business, it becomes very easy to see why being an effective communicator is vital to your own success.

There are many key ingredients placed into the pot of soup that eventually produces a great communicator. I would like to go over this recipe with you in some detail.

Know Your Subject Matter

Knowing your subject matter very well is the first criteria that must be satisfied if you are going to communicate an idea effectively. You must have complete control of the topic you are discussing and then you must be able to present your subject matter in a clear and logical manner to the targeted audience. The size of the audience can vary from one person to three hundred people in an auditorium setting. The size of the audience does not really matter as long as you are knowledgeable and logical in delivering the presentation.

Think Before Speaking

Always remember to think before you open your mouth. Once you say something, it is hard to take it back. You only get one shot at making the presentation to your audience and you do not want to blow that opportunity by blurting something out that you really did not mean to say.

Always Be Prepared

Take an adequate amount of time to prepare your presentations so that they come across in a completely professional manner. I have witnessed on more than a few occasions, chiropractic interns who were quite unprepared to give an official report of findings presentation to a patient. The students in these scenarios were constantly fumbling around for the right words to say, had x-rays that were not marked properly, and could not answer the patient's questions adequately. Most of these presentations turned out to be very unprofessional. Situations such as these can be avoided simply by taking a little time to make sure that you are prepared.

Listen Carefully

Learn to be a great listener. A big part of being a good communicator is having the ability to realize that communication is an exchange of ideas between two or more parties. You have to do some careful listening in order that you can eventually interject your own pearls of wisdom into a conversation. If everyone just concentrated on delivering ideas all the time and nobody ever took the time to do any listening we would have many situations where the lines of communication would constantly break down. Unfortunately this happens more often than people realize. Generally speaking most of us are not very good listeners and this makes it even more challenging for individuals trying to present information.

Be Confident

Be confident in what you are talking about. People can sense the confidence or the lack of confidence that you possess. Being confident is a direct product of being prepared, and knowing your subject. Sometimes nerves can get in the way and make it seem as if we are not prepared or confident while doing a presentation. A great way to overcome feelings of nervousness is to practice your presentations repeatedly while visualizing yourself in front of large numbers of people. If you do this exercise on a regular basis you will become much more relaxed during the live presentation.

Avoid Speaking in a Monotone Voice

Try not to speak in a monotone voice, as this will most likely put your audience into a hypnotic trance. Practice speaking with a voice tone that will vary throughout your entire presentation. Remember to try and keep the changes in your voice tone consistent with the body of information you are discussing at any given time. The intonation of a speaker's voice is going to be a key factor in the audience's level of comprehension in regards to the subject matter you are trying to present.

Do Not Stretch the Truth

Never stretch the truth when trying to communicate information to others. Be truthful and never tell a lie. A lie or information included in your presentation that is not completely accurate can come back to haunt you in many ways. These types of scenarios can undermine your credibility for the remainder of your professional career.

Keep it Simple

One of the most valuable things I have discovered over the years that I have been a practicing chiropractor is that it is a good policy to keep concepts very simple when trying to convey a point to patients. Laypersons really do not care to hear about all of the technical information you learned in college. In many instances, patients will just want the chiropractor to perform his or her technique so they can get back to their busy schedules.

I am constantly telling students that once they graduate from chiropractic college they will need to relearn the English language in order to be able to converse with their patients. I often overhear chiropractic interns instructing patients to lie on the adjusting tables in a supine or prone position. The patients often look at the students in a puzzled manner. Eventually the interns will realize what has happened and they will give their instructions once again telling the patients to lie face up or face down on the table.

Be Positive

When speaking or writing try to keep the information in a positive light. Even if the material you are presenting is negative in nature, there are clever ways that you can put a positive spin on the situation.

Adding humor to your presentation is very acceptable and also an excellent way to keep your audience from feeling depressed about material that might be perceived as slightly negative or somewhat depressing. Get creative and do not limit your ideas to just the ones presented here.

Be Natural

Be yourself! Stay within the boundaries of your own personality and you will be fine. Do not try to pass yourself off as someone you are not. This is a recipe for disaster and people will sense right away that you are not a sincere person.

Nervous Tics

Try to eliminate nervous tics and any other unpleasant body gestures that you might not be aware of. If you are constantly doing these bad habits on a regular basis your audience might become distracted and not pay attention to the content of your presentation. I would suggest you have a friend videotape some of the speaking presentations you perform so that you can analyze and remove any unusual habits that you might happen to observe.

Summarize Your Message

Remember to wrap up your presentation with a good summary. Summarizing the various concepts which you have discussed makes it easier for your audience to understand what exactly you want them to take away from the conversation. This is how you close the deal. Your ability to provide a first class summary about the key points covered in your material is going to go a long way in making the overall presentation a success.

Miscellaneous Forms of Communication

The miscellaneous forms of communication can be just as important in conveying a message as some of the other headings we have talked about. Little things are important, like maintaining healthy eye contact with your entire audience and not constantly staring at the same few people in the crowd. Facial expressions that give off an aura of your genuine sincerity will help draw people into your presentation. Body posture that supports an individual who is confident and excited about the information being presented along with a wardrobe that yells out how successful you are, can all be beneficial tools to help keep people tuned into what you are selling. Last but not least, I need to mention the importance of a good, old-fashioned hand shake between you and the members of your audience which immediately demonstrates that you are approachable, compassionate, and a concerned professional.

I cannot emphasize enough the importance of becoming an effective communicator. By following the advice offered in this chapter you will greatly improve your ability to communicate with patients and staff members which will help you to accomplish your primary objective of becoming a successful chiropractor.

4

Never Compromise Your Principles

4

Never Compromise Your Principles

One of the most important things you must learn in this lifetime is that there are certain universal truths that are self-evident and unchangeable. When you become mature enough to recognize what these truths are, you will be faced with having to make an important decision about whether or not you will incorporate these universal truths into your own life. Many people before you have had to think long and hard about the same, tough decision. You will have two options to consider. You can embrace these truths and accept them into your life, or you can settle for something that is less than the truth. Before making your final decision you should remember that anything less than the truth is known as a compromise.

The fourth secret to becoming a successful chiropractor is to find that magical set of principles that you can live by. Although these principles might not be the same for each and every person, they are, without a doubt, a major factor and a driving force in the lives of most people who aspire to be successful.

Once you are able to identify the principles that make up the driving force within your own life, make sure that you never compromise such principles for any reason whatsoever. Materialistic props have been used repeatedly during the course of our history to try and convince people to give up the strong principles they have stood for. This practice is very much a part of our own modern society and is an ugly blemish on the face of our nation's healthcare industry.

Over the years the profession of chiropractic has had many of its doctors attacked and coerced into compromising their principles. These assaults have been engineered by individuals, committees, agencies, lobbyists, lawmakers, unions, petrochemical corporations, and global elitists who have worked exceedingly hard to try and break the strong resolve of many men and women. Despite the continuous assaults on these doctors over an extended period of years the chiropractic profession has managed to survive.

Those of us who have had a glimpse of just how rough the waters within this profession have been are often amazed that there is even a profession called chiropractic still operating. A lot of money has been spent over the years, by extremely powerful organizations, in an attempt to quell the principles that the profession is based upon. In spite of numerous attacks that have been financed by transnational corporations that do not want chiropractic principles being promoted throughout mainstream America, chiropractic continues to exist and the primary reason is because chiropractic is based largely on a set of iron clad universal truths.

All of the money in the world cannot kill a universal truth. You might be able to suppress a few of them for lengthy periods of time but eventually the truths will resurface once again. In a nutshell, the chiropractic practice goal of correcting vertebral subluxations allows a better expression of health in the human body. Because this practice goal is based on a number of universal truths and there are many people who understand the value of these principles in maintaining a person's health, there will always be individuals in the world trying to practice this healthcare objective. In the future these people may not be called chiropractors and perhaps they will not be able to legally practice this objective in a particular country. In the end this will not matter and the practice objective will survive the annals of time regardless of man's artificial laws.

Successful chiropractors are a unique collection of men and women who are able to live comfortably within the parameters of a finite number of universal truths. They understand the value of knowing about these truths and are usually successful in many areas of their lives because of their abilities to stick with such principles.

It is easy to go with the flow, follow the crowd, and generally stay within the boundaries of conventionality. Many people in the world are not bothered by having to accept something that is less than the truth. They have been conditioned by society that it is okay to accept the concept of compromise. It is acceptable to these individuals to give up what they truly believe in. In exchange for such a compromise, they have been offered materialistic rewards. It happens all the time and after a while a person becomes numb and quite unaware of the damage this does to their soul.

I have spoken to a large number of chiropractors throughout my career who have made this compromise. These doctors have given up their sound principles and an understanding of what they knew to be logical truths just so they could become compliant with the dictates of a society that demanded as much. Why would an intelligent person do such a thing? What kind of societal pressures would cause someone to give up their strong convictions about something as important as a universal truth? I cannot answer these questions because in my opinion, there is not an answer that makes sense. It is one thing to practice something that goes against logic and truth because you have been the recipient of inaccurate information. It is another thing, and quite disturbing to observe the same behavior pattern in individuals who have access to the logical principles yet still choose to settle for something that is less than the truth.

A Personal Story

Many years ago I had a friend who asked me to become involved with a company that sold a line of skin care products. I told my friend on a number of occasions that I was not really interested in getting involved with this sort of business. I was busy with my own private practice and did not want to lose focus of my personal goals. After much persistence, and because this fellow was a friend, I agreed to pay the minimal investment and I became affiliated with this company.

The business plan of the *XYZ Company* (not the real company name) called for the investors involved to spend a great deal of time trying to sell the actual business opportunity to other prospective investors. It became blatantly obvious to me after just a few days of being involved with this organization that my own future success within this company was going to be determined by my ability to sell the business opportunity to others and that the skin care product was pretty much an afterthought in the minds of most of the business partners.

I did a little research on the *XYZ Company* and found out that the marketing strategy they were utilizing was called "*multi-level-marketing.*" I also uncovered some additional information and found out that there were a couple of very successful companies that existed within the United States that employed this type of marketing system. Originally I was very suspicious of the *XYZ Company* and real curious to see if the business opportunity was legal. I can assure you that I am not a lawyer and I am not an expert in legal issues. Nevertheless, I convinced myself that this company I was involved with was in fact operating on the proper side of the law.

To make a long story somewhat shorter let me just tell you that I lost interest in attending the company's required weekly meetings. Within less than a month I became an inactive member of the organization. About three months later my friend quit the company as well and we never talked about this lost business opportunity or the topic of *"multi-level- marketing"* ever again.

About two years later I met a man who became a regular patient in my private practice. We became friendly and shared some personal insights on business ventures. Fred Smith (not his real name) was a very wealthy individual and I learned that he had made a large chunk of his money in a *"multi-level-marketing"* company. Fred was earning a large monthly income from a business that was similar to the one I had been involved with a couple of years earlier. I asked Fred one evening about his company and the marketing system that it used and he proceeded to tell me why only a few companies had ever managed to be successful in using such a system.

The secret, as it turned out, was plain old common sense and I should have realized this years earlier when I was involved with the *XYZ Company*. Fred's company was built around a super product that people desired on a regular basis. This company was very service-oriented and their mission statement was built on realistic goals and sound business principles. The major focus of Fred's company was centered on selling the product and not the business opportunity. The company was based on logical business truths and the marketing system (the vehicle chosen to drive the business) worked because it was attached to a company that would not under any circumstances compromise their principles. Enough said!

I know that I went off on a tangent with the last story, but I thought that it very clearly demonstrated a practical example of the major point I have been stressing in this chapter. The point being that successful people always stick with the principles they know and believe in. When you deviate from the truth you are basically setting yourself up for future failure. Always try to be true to your cause and offer no amount of flexibility when it comes to your principles or beliefs.

Whether we are talking about a chiropractic practice, a *"multi-level-marketing"* company, or the personal philosophy which we use on an everyday basis to navigate through the obstacle course commonly referred to as life, it is important to be true to your heart. The materialistic props that are tempting to all human beings must be carefully weighed and kept in proper perspective. Money and material items are a necessity in our world however; one must carefully consider what he or she is willing to sell. Hopefully the principles which are the driving force behind your own life are not included on a list of items that you are willing to sell.

5

Believe in the Value
of the Service you Perform

5

Believe in the Value
of the Service you Perform

The fifth secret to becoming a successful chiropractor is one of the most overlooked ingredients of the entire formula. Every practicing chiropractor who has a desire to be successful needs to believe wholeheartedly in the value of the service he or she is performing.

It is virtually impossible to sell a product or a service to someone if the person doing the selling is not convinced that the product or service being offered for sale is valuable and worth the asking price. There are countless numbers of chiropractors in our profession who do not believe their services are very valuable. Many of these doctors are hesitant to ask patients for payments when services have been rendered. Some doctors will even allow patients to manage their own care.

I personally have no trouble whatsoever believing in the value of the chiropractic service I perform for my patients. Throughout my career as a practicing chiropractor there have been a few isolated occasions where a patient has asked me to justify my professional fees. I can remember quite vividly the very first time this happened and how I responded to the inquiry. After recovering from the initial shock of the patient asking me such a direct question, I quickly explained to the individual that my professional service was so valuable that very few people in the community would be able to afford it. I made it very clear that because I was in the healthcare business and had a genuine concern for my patients' well-being, I felt compelled to set a professional fee which was realistic for people of all income brackets.

Doctors who believe in the value of the chiropractic service they are performing will automatically gain enormous confidence when making professional decisions for their patients. Suddenly, the little things that once stressed out these practitioners, such as asking patients to pay their fees while maintaining a suggested visit frequency, are no longer a concern.

You need to ask yourself if you believe in the value of the service you perform. Do you live the philosophy you preach? Are you under chiropractic care getting your own spine checked on a regular basis? Would you pay for this service if you had to? These are all very important questions that you will need to answer at some point. The answers that you come up with will ultimately give you the answer to the bigger and more important question that needs to be addressed which is whether or not you place any real value in the professional service you are currently administering. If you find out that you do not value the service you provide, you will have identified a very serious problem that will need some immediate attention.

It is important to remember that although the chiropractor sets the professional fee in his or her office, it is the patient who determines the actual value of the service. The patient will directly determine the value of a given service by assessing information that is derived directly from the chiropractor.

The following items represent a list of practice behaviors which are commonly observed in chiropractic offices where the doctors do not value the services they regularly perform. If these behaviors are present in your own office this is a clear signal to your patients that you do not value the service you are providing for them.

Practice Behaviors That Lower the Value of the Chiropractic Service You Perform

1. I let my patients decide when to come in for care.

2. I do not hold my patients accountable for co-payments and deductibles.

3. I never hold my patients accountable for missed appointments.

4. I do not make an attempt to educate patients about the benefits of chiropractic care for other family members and friends.

5. I do not ask my patients for referrals.

6. I avoid talking to patients about additional exams or services they may need.

7. I am always willing to lower my professional fees just so the patient will not go to another office.

8. I do not provide my own family members with regular chiropractic care.

9. I am not under chiropractic care.

In the final analysis you must have a tremendous amount of confidence in the service you offer. You must believe that chiropractic care will be beneficial for all of your patients. You have to be able to express this confidence at all times and your patients and staff members have to understand that your service is valuable as well.

If you can believe that what you do is worth while you will have the energy and confidence to show others how to benefit from your service and you will be successful in selling your service to anyone who enters your practice.

6

Avoid Burnout

6

Avoid Burnout

The sixth secret to becoming a successful chiropractor is to avoid professional burnout. The same attributes that can help an individual to become successful in life can also be the key factors in causing the person to become frustrated and filled with emotions of depression and despair. It is important to realize that your life is made up of many different parts and that in order for you to be happy and successful you will need to create some sort of balance between these parts.

Many professionals who are goal-oriented, run into the trap of working themselves into a state of physical and emotional burnout. I am not a psychologist who specializes in this sort of disorder, however I have had an opportunity in my own life to experience firsthand the effects of professional burnout.

In order to avoid periods of burnout, which can be very destructive to your own life, you must be able to recognize the various indicators that often accompany this condition. Most of us have probably heard the saying *"The first step in solving a problem is identifying one."* I often wonder if people realize how accurate this statement is. A large number of people who suffer from emotional and physical burnout are not even aware that they have such problems. The condition pretty much sneaks up on them while they are busy living their lives. All of a sudden they are in trouble and in need of help. Unfortunately, in many instances, help is not available and the people doing the suffering have absolutely nowhere to turn.

Some of the indicators of this condition are discussed below. If you are able to identify any of these items in your own life it might be a good idea for you to pay very close attention to the material contained in this chapter.

Obviously, symptomatic indicators can vary in their intensities and this author is not trying to offer a treatment plan or to provide a specific diagnosis for individuals. This information is to be used for educational purposes only and should not be misinterpreted, by the reader, as a substitute for a proper psychological evaluation by a qualified professional.

Feelings of Frustration

One of the most common indicators of work-related burnout is the presence of frustration within your life. No matter what it is you are trying to accomplish, there will be this overwhelming feeling that some divine force is trying to impede your progress. Feelings of frustration can manifest in your professional life at the onset of this disorder and then later on will begin to show up in your personal and family life as well.

Daydreaming

Very often, people who are suffering from the effects of burnout will spend a good portion of their time thinking about alternative life or job related scenarios that might be perceived by such individuals as being less stressful or perhaps even more exciting than their current life situations. Daydreaming is often utilized by those of us who are suffering from burnout because it provides a temporary form of escapism from various sets of circumstances that have caused problems to take shape in the first place. Professionals who regularly daydream about changes in their lifestyle could quite possibly be suffering from a form of work related burnout.

Physical and Mental Exhaustion

Another indicator that is often reported by workers plagued with burnout is their constant feelings of being exhausted, no matter how much sleep they are able to acquire. In this situation the persons suffering with these problems will often try to work through the apparent feelings of fatigue only to discover that their physical and mental exhaustion never seems to leave them.

Emotional Meltdowns

Burnout will very often cause individuals to suddenly and without warning develop unusual feelings that directly lead to emotional outbursts or fits of rage. These emotional meltdowns, are in many situations, uncontrollable as well as completely unpredictable. The slightest little event could cause sufferers to "snap" into an episode for no apparent reason.

Emotional outbursts can cause many problems in the workplace environment and can eventually feed into the original problem by creating more frustration and an even deeper state of burnout.

Feelings of Depression and Despair

Some of the most intense symptomatic indicators of burnout experienced by persons in the workplace are continuous feelings of depression along with the prevailing attitude that there is little chance for any help within the immediate future. Feelings of this nature can be so strong that some people experiencing such emotions often consider drastic actions.

Feelings of Negativity

Strong feelings of negativity will often be present in people who suffer from burnout. Almost everything that these individuals are associated with becomes bathed in an attitude of doom and gloom. Professionals who are usually upbeat and very positive in their daily interactions with patients and staff members are suddenly a cancer within their own businesses. The strong, negative vibrations these people are harboring are immediately perceived by practice members and the effects of the overall situation are quickly revealed by a number of practice statistics which will additionally confirm the presence of a problem over time.

Panic Attacks

Shortness of breath, pain in your chest, a rapid heart beat, indigestion, fatigue, and a feeling of impending doom that is lurking over you are just a few of the symptoms associated with having a panic attack. Numerous people in the world suffer from panic disorders or similar stress-related episodes. It would be inaccurate to report that all of these panic disorder cases are directly attributed to a specific category of work-related stress. However, it is certainly plausible and a working hypothesis of many psychologists that a substantial number of these cases are a direct result of pressures in the workplace. Keep in mind that many individuals suffering from professional and work-related burnout are prone to having panic attacks.

Increased Appetite

The cumulative effect of these indicators will often cause an individual to experience an increase in his or her appetite. All of a sudden the routine of eating more food helps to soothe the pain that is being caused by the large number of problems that we have been discussing. Obviously increased appetite will eventually lead to excessive weight gain which often reinforces feelings of guilt and even more depression. These indicators all seem to feed off of one another and become part of a great big vicious cycle that is very difficult to break away from.

It Happened to Me

I like to think of myself as an optimistic person who is able to pick out the smallest components representing something positive in an otherwise very bleak situation. I have always positioned my emotional tuner at a setting which was compatible with picking up vibrations that were resonating at higher and more positive frequency ranges.

In the late 90s, I experienced a severe case of work-related burnout. It was at this time that I became inundated with extreme feelings of negativity that I had not previously experienced. These feelings were obviously triggered by my own obsessive work habits which caused me to experience many of the indicators of burnout that I have been writing about in this chapter. Although this was a very short period of time in my life, it turned out to be a very costly experience from a financial point of view.

As a result of my emotional state of mind, during those couple of years, I made decisions to walk away from two, very lucrative professional practices that I had built from the ground up and to move to an entirely new state in order to begin a career as a college instructor. The negativity which I had experienced during this time of my life as well as my decision to leave my private practice was not very representative of my overall personality. These two decisions however, offered me an opportunity to make necessary changes in my life that would eventually allow me the time to rest and recover from the problems I had been suffering from. As it turned out these decisions would be the most important ones I have ever made. They ultimately gave me an opportunity to balance out those other parts of my life which had been neglected for so many years. The financial loss I experienced, that seemed somewhat traumatic at the time, was a sacrifice I needed to make in order to get my life back on track. A few years later I was able to recover from my financial woes and suddenly the pain in my wallet magically disappeared. I realize today that the financial concerns that had once been a part of my life were much easier to correct than some of the problems which were affecting my overall health and well being. Given the same identical set of circumstances I would have to make the same decisions all over again. It was the only way that I could have successfully solved the emotional and physical burnout which I was experiencing at the time.

Preventing Burnout

There are a number of proactive steps that you can take to prevent these problems. Again it is important to remember that recognition of key indicators can be helpful in solving a situation before it has the chance to manifest into an absolutely full blown disorder that might require professional help. Here are some helpful ideas for preventing burnout.

Pace Yourself

One of the most important things I have learned so far is how to create a healthy pace within my own work environment. This allows me the luxury of getting an objective completed without placing too much stress on my psyche. When you learn how to adhere to a healthy pace in your own life this will do wonders for you.

If you think about this logically, it makes perfect sense. Imagine for a moment about how a long distance runner and a sprinter prepare for a competition. Both athletes compete in track events that require a different pace. If the two athletes did not have any idea about how far they would have to run they would have a difficult time becoming successful in each of their events. The pace that is used by the sprinter is certainly going to be different than the pace that is utilized by the long distance runner. Having a proper pace will ensure the two runners a better chance of success within their given categories of competition. The same logic can and should be applied when tackling projects in the workplace.

Allow Time for Rest and Relaxation

It is easy to let yourself become obsessed with a work project. Having proper amounts of time set aside for periods of rest and relaxation will be quite helpful in keeping you fresh and recharged for when you do return to your place of business.

Rest and relaxation does not mean that you should just sit on the couch in front of the television set for a couple of hours. Periods of rest and relaxation must have a definite quality built into them. Learn how to take vacations and get yourself away from daily routines. A change of scenery can also be helpful in becoming more relaxed. Even two or three day excursions to new destinations can be helpful in breaking the rut and boredom of the everyday grind. Remember that you work very hard for a living so it is important that you reward yourself during the year with multiple opportunities to get away from the workplace.

When you are on vacation do not take your cell phone or pager with you. If you take these items on a vacation, you are actually taking your work with you and you are not really removing yourself from the office. Make arrangements for someone to fill in for you at your practice or shut the doors for a couple of days. Get your patients comfortable with the idea that you need to be sharp while working with them and in order to be at your best you need to rest and relax like anybody else. Do not be ashamed of taking time off from work so that you can go on a vacation. Practice good rest and relaxation habits and you will stay excited and fresh in the office for many years to come.

Spend Quality Time With Your Family

It is extremely important that you spend quality time with your spouse and children. I believe that a successful marriage is an important prerequisite for having a happy and successful practice. Once again I will try to impress upon you the necessity of creating balance between these two aspects of your life. I honestly believe that many chiropractors get so wrapped up in their passion for the profession that they often neglect the most important people in their lives – family members. Keeping careful focus on the big picture of life and making sure that your domestic affairs are in order will go a long way in helping you to accomplish the professional goals you set out to achieve.

It is not very realistic for chiropractors to believe that they will have success in running a professional practice if in fact they constantly stumble in their attempts to have successful personal relationships. These two components of our lives are quite interrelated and will regularly impact one another. Practitioners who become aware of the connection between the two components early in their careers are usually the doctors who are also successful in their practice lives.

Celebrate the Goals You Achieve

In an earlier chapter I wrote about creating realistic goals. The point that I wanted to highlight in this chapter is that many frustrations as well as other emotional problems that are commonly observed as a result of work related stress can be avoided altogether by simply making sure that the goals you set are kept realistic enough so you can achieve them.

Once you do achieve a goal do not be afraid to celebrate the accomplishment. Take the time to reward yourself for all the hard work that you have performed. Make sure that you celebrate these accomplishments with your spouse and children who are your support team. Acknowledging the completion of one goal will also help you to focus more clearly on the next objective on your list of priorities.

Have a Hobby

Having a hobby or an interest in a particular area that exists outside of your chosen profession is a great idea. People who devote all of their energy and spare time to the workplace are setting themselves up for problems.

I have always maintained a variety of hobbies which I like to devote time to. I am a chiropractor and college instructor by trade but my professional resume does not make up my entire life. Although chiropractic is very important to me, it is by no means the only interest within my life. I have many hobbies that lie outside the lines of the chiropractic profession. These hobbies allow me to keep my professional life exciting. I do not become bored with my profession because I have learned to live with it harmoniously and

I have learned to leave it on the shelf, at times, when I am doing something I enjoy which is outside of my professional life. I implore you to do the same in your own life.

7

Do Not Fear Success

7

Do Not Fear Success

I once knew a patient who was a fabulous artist. This woman could paint absolutely anything she desired. Her ability to create a scene on a previously blank piece of canvas just amazed me. I always imagined she would make it to the top within her field. I also remember that this woman was never satisfied with any of the paintings she would produce. She was always trying to tweak her creations so they would be more professional-looking in their appearance.

One day I asked her why she never tried to sell any of her paintings in the commercial markets. She told me that although her work was good it could be much better. She also claimed to be a perfectionist and wanted her productions to be flawless before putting them up for sale.

Over the few years that I took care of this patient she never did sell any of her paintings despite the fact that they were all absolutely magnificent works of art. I always believed that this patient, deep down inside, was intentionally trying to obstruct her own potential success. She always seemed to find a convenient excuse which would help rescue her from having to sell her paintings. In my opinion she was absolutely terrified of becoming successful within her field.

The seventh secret to becoming a successful chiropractor is to make sure you do not fear the various rewards that might come into your own life as a result of your professional accomplishments. Many professionals in our society have a terrible fear of becoming successful in a particular area of their lives and subconsciously try to impede their own efforts to accomplish objectives or goals.

You might question why a person would be afraid of his or her own success. At face value it does seem like a very strange phobia. Nevertheless, there are quite a few professionals in the world who wrestle with these types of challenges.

With success comes the status and reputation of being a winner. When you become a winner, the pressures to maintain a certain level of excellence can become immense. In many situations the pressures to stay on top are too much for certain individuals to handle and so they choose to remove themselves from the spotlight. Other reasons that professionals are afraid of success are listed as follows:

Other Reasons Professionals Are Afraid of Success

1. Some professionals lack confidence and suffer from very low self-esteem.

2. Some professionals are afraid of the limelight that will be generated from achieving success.

3. Some professionals are afraid of the jealousy that will come from colleagues within their industry.

4. Some professionals are afraid that their successful status will suddenly become compromised or withdrawn.

5. Some professionals are afraid that once they attain a certain level of success they will begin a downward spiral in their careers due to a lack of desire to work on future goals.

How I developed a Healthy Attitude About Being Successful

As a child I was regularly involved with organized sports. The many scenarios which I had a chance to experience while taking part in competitive events offered me a wonderful opportunity to develop positive life skills that I have been able to apply to different areas of my professional life. I learned very early in my childhood how becoming a champion was a label which brought many responsibilities and pressures that were basically nonexistent prior to attaining such a level of success.

At a young age, thirteen other boys and I were fortunate enough to experience a wonderful summer of baseball that culminated in winning a Little League World Championship in Williamsport, Pennsylvania. I was able to experience during the summer months of 1975 what most people will never experience in their entire lives. I was able to play for and win a world championship on national television. This experience provided me with a number of pressures and responsibilities that young children normally do not have to deal with. I learned very early in my life what the words success and responsibility really meant.

When you win a world championship at age twelve you become a marked person—a target for others to conquer. As strange as this may seem, it is absolutely the truth. Throughout the remainder of my childhood career in organized sports there was a tremendous amount of animosity that was projected in my direction from others who were quite envious of the Little League experience I had taken part in. Because I was forced, as a child, to deal with various jealousies and competitive situations that were placed on my doorstep, I was able to gain tremendous insight, knowledge, and strength on how to handle success and the pressures attached to that word. As a result of the unusual amount of success I was exposed to as a child, it has been much easier for me in my adult years to set personal and professional goals and to accept success whenever I was able to achieve it.

Having a healthy attitude about becoming successful and learning how to deal with the side items that are served up as a result of achieving success are important lessons to learn. You will need to have a very healthy attitude about achieving success if you want to remain at a particular level of excellence once you complete an objective.

I believe that it is extremely important for chiropractors to remain highly motivated once they have managed to succeed in a particular area of their lives. If a doctor practices certain techniques which ensure his or her eventual success in completing an objective it would not be very logical for that person to eliminate those tools of success once the objective has been reached.

It is equally important to remember that you have to be thick-skinned in life. You cannot spend valuable time worrying about hypothetical remarks of a negative nature that are supposedly coming from colleagues and other professionals. By keeping your attitude healthy and your goals within close range you will not have time to worry about these unhealthy distractions. In the end it will be you and you alone who will ultimately determine whether or not you embrace success in a healthy manner.

8

Create a Patient Referral Program

8

Create a Patient Referral Program

Every chiropractor would like to know the magical secret to bringing lots of new patients into his or her private office setting. The secret is actually not that complicated and certainly very easy to implement into any professional practice. The first thing you will need to do is to come to terms with the fact that the chiropractic profession usually does not receive much in the way of cooperative advertising from the media or other health related fields. In other words you are not going to get a tremendous amount of help in building your practice from outside sources. If you want to build a large patient base, you are going to have to do this task on your own.

The eighth secret to becoming a successful chiropractor is to make sure that you create an efficient patient referral program that will ensure your practice receives a constant stream of new patients on a regular basis. You will need to teach your patients the importance of referring others for professional services.

Earlier in this book I discussed the importance of becoming an effective communicator. This skill will be utilized often when building your patient referral system.

You will need to teach already existing patients how to properly refer new prospects into your office. You will do this simply by teaching your practice members the importance of chiropractic care for the entire family. Let your existing patients know that chiropractic is a valuable service for all people who have a desire to be healthy. Existing patients will also need to be able to understand simple chiropractic principles and, more importantly, they must be able to convey the principles to other lay persons within the community.

Fortunately, most of the principles that laypersons will need to learn in order to regularly refer patients into your office are very simple concepts to understand. Make sure that you keep these concepts simple when presenting them to your patients. Resist the urge to make things more complicated than they need to be when going through your explanations with patients. It is human nature to take something that is very simple and to make it more complex. If you do this you will not have a successful referral campaign.

Teach the Five Concepts

The first concept you will need to teach to patients is how the body is always trying to maintain itself in a healthy state of existence. Give an explanation on how the body does everything in its power to keep itself healthy and how in situations where it has become compromised by sickness it will do everything possible to try and restore order.

The second concept you will need to teach to patients is how health is maintained naturally with the help of the human nervous system. Explain to your patients how the brain, spinal cord, and spinal nerves help to transmit electrical messages *(instructions for health)* to all areas of the body and that this ultimately ensures health in human beings.

The third concept you will teach to your patients is how the spinal bones protect the nervous system from detrimental external forces while simultaneously allowing humans the ability to move around with a great deal of agility.

The fourth concept you must teach to your patients is how misalignments of the spinal bones (subluxations) can interfere with the delivery and transmission of the electrical messages inside the nervous system. You must teach patients that the normal tendencies for the body to be healthy are largely dependent on these electrical messages being transmitted through the nervous system properly and without any interference.

The fifth and final concept you must teach to your patients is how a chiropractic spinal adjustment is capable of correcting a subluxation within the spinal column. You need patients to understand that when a subluxation is removed from the equation the interference within the nervous system is eliminated and this allows the body to express itself once again in a healthy manner.

These concepts will appear quite logical to laypersons the very first time they have a chance to hear them. If they are presented properly by the chiropractor to already existing patients, it will not take very long for those patients to be able to relate the chiropractic story to other laypersons within the community. This can be a very powerful referral tool for your practice once you learn how to utilize the system properly.

Create an Incentive Plan

The next thing you must do is to create an incentive plan for your patients to go out and sell your service. Some of your patients will become motivated to generate referrals for your practice just from their understanding of these five chiropractic concepts and they will not require an incentive from you to get the job done. You should be prepared however to offer the patients in your practice some kind of an incentive to ensure the program's success. You need to understand that most people enjoy recognition for a job that has been competently performed. My suggestion is that you thank your patients on a regular basis for the referrals which they send to your office. Saying thank you to a patient that is helping you to build your practice is easy. A handshake, a post card in the mail, an email communication on the Internet, a message board featuring the patient's name and accomplishment posted in a conspicuous location within your office are very acceptable ways to thank patients. In addition to saying thank you it wouldn't hurt to reward patients with an occasional gift certificate to a movie theatre or to a popular department store. Perhaps you might even consider issuing a t-shirt, which advertises your practice, to the patient who generates the most referrals within a given month. *(Make sure you check with your state's chiropractic board to see if a particular incentive reward is legal.)*

Helpful Tools

There are a number of very good chiropractic books on the market that have been specifically written to teach laypersons important chiropractic principles. In 2002 I personally authored the book *"Chiropractic Made Simple: Working With the Controlling Laws of Nature" PageFree Publishing, Inc.* This book can be purchased from Amazon.com as well as from many other Internet book distributors around the world. I highly recommend that you have your patients read this text at some point. *"Chiropractic Made Simple"* teaches patients the importance of wellness care and it also teaches patients the importance of referring others. Many chiropractors in the United States now require their new patients to read this book before getting under care.

Keep in mind that incentive-based referral programs are very well received in the chiropractic office environment. If structured properly the existing patients within your private practice will regularly generate hundreds of new patient referrals on an annual basis. In the end this will allow you to focus more of your attention on helping your patients.

Outside marketing procedures will probably continue to be a necessary part of your overall practice building strategies; however the pressures to bring in newer prospects via the use of external campaigns will be significantly reduced once you implement this type of a program.

9

Manage Time Efficiently

9

Manage Time Efficiently

The ninth secret to becoming a successful chiropractor is to make sure that you learn to manage time efficiently. You need to make an effort, on a regular basis, to notice how you are spending time in both your personal and professional lives.

Many people often find out that they are not being as effective as they could be with their own time management procedures. There are certain events that regularly occur during the course of a day which will cause individuals to become distracted from what they are trying to accomplish. One of the many things I learned as a practicing chiropractor was how to identify daily distractions which were preventing my own productivity. With a little bit of practice and a lot of concentration I was able to identify "chunks of clutter" that were causing major distractions in my life and needed to be thrown away.

Clean Out Your Garage

A few years ago my wife and I decided to undertake a major project in our home. We began to clean out our garage and throw away many older items which we had accumulated over the years. This was a chore we had been putting off for quite some time. Even though we were aware of the fact that we needed to get this job done, we still managed to find a variety of excuses to defer the project to a much later date.

Our garage was littered with contents that neither one of us had touched for several years. We had conveniently stacked many of these items which we no longer seemed to have a need for in various locations throughout the garage. Because of all the clutter, we were unable to garage our cars, lawnmowers, yard tools, and other contents which we regularly used. Our garage was completely non-functional due to all of the trash we had collected.

Finally after a lot of procrastination, we tackled the project and began to take back our space. Once we finished the job we both felt very positive about what we had accomplished. We were now able to use this part of our house once again. With all of the old junk conveniently removed and out of the way, we had access to many tools that had been previously hidden. It was great to have our garage space in such an organized state. I now looked forward to walking inside my garage once again while looking for various tools that I needed for jobs around the house. Prior to our cleaning up this disaster, I did not have the urge to walk through this area. If I needed to get something in the garage I instantly became disgusted from observing all of the items that had been thrown around.

The cleaning project my wife and I accomplished demonstrates what can happen to people when they allow distractions in their lives, which should be discarded, to pile up. They become overwhelmed with the distractions and this prevents these individuals from becoming efficient managers of time.

In order to be a good manager of time you will need to clean out the junk in your own life and become very organized. When an individual has a neat working environment and is very organized he or she is more likely to plan things out in a logical manner. Organization skills can help a person eliminate wasted procedures which are often costly for those of us who consider time a very precious commodity.

Some Simple Advice

I have spoken with quite a few successful doctors over the years and many of these people have recommended the same logical advice over and over again. The advice is quite simple and calls for the professional to learn how to eliminate the various distractions which can occur in one's life. Additionally, I have attended numerous time management seminars during my career as a chiropractor. Many of the seminar speakers convey similar messages as well. The prevailing idea is that you need to figure out in advance the time of the day that you are getting most of your work accomplished. Once you have this time frame figured out you need to set up some solid ground rules which will prevent you from becoming disturbed during these productive hours.

One easy way that you can prevent distractions in your professional life is by delegating some of the work in your office to others. Let your chiropractic assistant or receptionist run interference for you while you tackle the more important tasks on the daily agenda. By utilizing your office staff you can take away some of the inherent pressures that are present in the work environment. Regular interruptions by solicitors, attorneys, patients, and many other sources can be screened and then deflected by a receptionist. This will ultimately allow the chiropractor to manage his or her time more efficiently.

Another wonderful tool which can help a professional to manage time efficiently is the utilization of a modern computer. Computers can cut down the amount of time that needs to be spent in preparing patient files, insurance claims, narrative reports, newsletters, and other office related chores. Many of us have grown up in an era when computers were non-existent. Because we are not always familiar with how some of these gadgets operate, we sometimes ignore the benefits which they might offer to our practices. It is probably a very good idea for chiropractors to invest both the time and money to purchase a computer along with an adequate training program that will teach doctors how to operate the equipment. In the long run an investment such as this might save a doctor quite a bit of money and more importantly – a lot of time.

Avoid Procrastination

Never put off until tomorrow what needs to be accomplished

right now. Procrastination is not a quality that is going to help you to manage your time efficiently. A person who is a procrastinator is simply a lazy person. A lazy person does not want to invest the necessary amount of time required to become successful. If you are constantly avoiding work which needs to be completed you might be guilty of being a procrastinator in which case you will need to give yourself a kick in the pants. For every good excuse you can come up with that favors delaying an important project you can come up with an even better reason why you should get the job done right now. Get in the habit of taking care of business when it is right in front of you. Never take the lazy approach when running your business.

A Final Thought

Try to always practice or implement good time management skills. If you are able to eliminate unnecessary tasks in the workplace, you will see many dividends in the way of better overall work production. This will eventually lead to a more efficient running chiropractic practice as well as a very happy and successful chiropractor.

10

Remember to Have Fun

10

Remember to Have Fun

The tenth secret to becoming a successful chiropractor is to remember to have fun while running your practice. So many people in the world dislike their jobs and pretty much dread the time they spend earning a living. The average person will work five or six days a week and is awarded approximately two weeks of vacation leave each year. With every passing day, people are challenged to make ends meet in a society that makes such a task extremely difficult. Yet, most workers remain loyal to their employers because they want the security that is offered by these occupational relationships.

As a doctor of chiropractic you have the potential to help many patients enjoy a better quality of life. There are very few healthcare professionals in the world who can realistically stand up and take credit for removing a major form of interference from the human body's physiology. We chiropractors are truly blessed to be involved with such a wonderful trade and I am not exaggerating when I write about the tremendous amount of personal satisfaction that is often experienced by practicing members of our profession. This feeling of satisfaction is due to the positive results which we regularly observe while taking care of our patients. In all honesty I have to confess that receiving so much satisfaction on a regular basis is a lot of fun!

Having fun within your practice will be an important component of your own success as a chiropractor. Unlike many professions within healthcare, chiropractic is exciting and especially rewarding. Patients will respond positively to your care when their nervous systems are cleared of interferences originating from vertebral subluxations. Because there are so many benefits and opportunities that come along with being a chiropractor, it is very hard not to have fun in this profession.

Throughout my career, many patients have asked me why I am so passionate about what I do for a living. They want to know why I am still able to have fun after being involved with this line of work for so many years. My answer simply stated is that this is a way of life for me. Chiropractic is not just a job that I perform for a few hours each day. It is without a doubt a lifestyle that I happen to agree with. I have learned many important lessons about life because of my association with this healthcare profession. When you learn the truth about something it really sets you free. Chiropractic has allowed me the opportunity to see the truth in many healthcare issues and I now have a clearer understanding of how to approach these subjects when counseling patients and chiropractic students.

Are You Having Fun?

Do you enjoy your profession? Are you excited about becoming a chiropractor in the near future? Do you still have the energy and enthusiasm that you possessed ten years ago when you were in the planning stages of getting your office up and running? Are you having fun doing the everyday things in your life? These are all very important questions for students and chiropractors to ponder. If you answer "no" to any of these questions you should take a few moments to ask yourself why you are unable to have fun in your daily life. What are the hurdles preventing you from enjoying the fruits of your labor? Life is too short to be miserable. Perhaps you need to lighten up and start incorporating your wonderful sense of humor directly into your practice routine. Having a healthy sense of humor (at all times) is a very important ingredient in maintaining one's sanity at home and in the workplace. It also allows individuals the chance to have fun in any arena they happen to find themselves in.

Having Fun in the Workplace

I have had many enjoyable moments while fulfilling my duties as a member of the teaching faculty at Sherman College of Straight Chiropractic. Employment at the college has afforded me an unusual opportunity to experience a side of our profession that few doctors ever get a chance to witness. When I have been in the classroom setting or in the college's health center supervising chiropractic interns, I have observed talented men and women who were truly motivated about learning their craft.

Quite a few of the students I have interacted with on a regular basis have compared their chiropractic college experiences to that of being in the eye of an emotional hurricane. Their perceptions of the chiropractic education process were all very similar as they described a four-year period of time that featured a constant flow of stress coming from every direction imaginable. In addition to the constant academic pressures students face, many of these future chiropractors have personally told me on numerous occasions that they were flat broke and in debt up to their eyeballs. In addition to these problems, most of the students were facing many more responsibilities in their lives than ever before. Contrary to the beliefs of some professors residing within the academic world, a large percentage of the students I have conversed with were very much aware of both the professional and financial challenges that were directly ahead of them. In spite of such adverse conditions, these individuals continued to have a lot of fun during their college careers and a large number of chiropractic students were able to remain focused on their studies while providing excellent care for their patients in the college's health center.

I have often wondered why so many chiropractic students were able to have fun while learning about their chosen profession while many licensed and well-established chiropractors were unable to enjoy the art which they regularly performed for their own patients. I believe that the answer to this question lies in the students' commitment to remain loyal to a given set of principles which they believe in. Students will very rarely compromise the truths which they have learned in school. In the business world, veteran chiropractors are usually not as committed to these philosophical doctrines and are sometimes willing to accept a compromised version of important practice principles. This scenario can often lead to a condition I like to call *"professional dissatisfaction."* The level of *"professional dissatisfaction"* that a particular practitioner might experience from time to time is going to be pretty much determined by the degree of compromise the individual is willing to absorb. If the compromise continues for an extended period of time, established professionals can become dangerously frustrated and this will eventually cause the doctors involved to lose the important sense of excitement about their practices which is necessary to create a fun and successful work environment.

Understanding the Game

I believe that it is very important for chiropractors, as well as students of chiropractic, to understand the game in which they are involved. If you want to be able to score points so that you can become competitive and have a chance to do well within the game, you will need to know all of the applicable rules. You will also need to understand who has designed the game in the first place. Remember to keep your sense of humor nearby because you will need to access it on many occasions.

You register and give your consent to be a player in the game the very first day you enroll as a student in a chiropractic college. It does not matter which college you attend because every college must charge you a sizeable fee for tuition expenses. The cost of a chiropractic education has increased steadily over the past twenty years and there is no reason to believe that this trend will change anytime soon.

The more debt that you create during your career as a student the worse your position on the game board will be once you finish school. Those students who graduate college with the most debt are immediately assigned the worst possible location on the game board. Obviously, the less debt that you accumulate as a student the better your assigned position will be when you become an active player in the game after your graduation. For those of you who are thinking that you have already destroyed your chances to do well in the game you should take a deep breath and relax. Most people in the chiropractic profession do not even realize that such a game exists. You can regularly improve your positioning within the game over time and doctors who have already graduated with minimal debt can make critical mistakes within their businesses and freefall to a lesser position on the game board. Just knowing that the game exists in the first place is going to give you an unbelievable advantage over other people playing in the contest.

Learning the rules of the game is essential to becoming successful within both the game and your practice. If you are playing basketball and you are trying to score points by throwing a football for touchdowns, you are going to have a lot of trouble scoring points. You have to know what sport you are involved in and you have to learn the objective of the sport so you know how to develop a proper strategy so that you will eventually be able to score some serious points.

The Designers of the Game

The designers of the game are the transnational petrochemical corporations that pretty much control the world of healthcare. They control a lot of other things besides healthcare but that is an entirely different area of discussion that I will address later on in this book.

The petrochemical corporations own the pharmaceutical companies, the insurance companies, the hospitals, the health practitioners, the accrediting agencies, the licensing boards and pretty much anything else which exists that is a form of valuable property or is considered to be an asset within the world healthcare arena.

The game has been designed, not for your entertainment, but rather for the purpose of securing you as an asset that will also be owned by the transnational petrochemical corporations of the world. This is not a joke and I am not kidding about the existence of the game or the planned servitude these companies have set aside for you and others within the chiropractic profession.

The Game Begins

The game begins to heat up once you have graduated from a chiropractic college. You now have a rather large sum of money (your student loan) which you must begin to pay back to the government. You have come out of school as a principled chiropractor (the principles may be different for each individual) and you enter the business world trying to set up a practice so that you can make a difference in the lives of your patients. Equipped with your principles you start out with the best of intentions. What you soon begin to realize is that it will be very hard for you to make enough money to pay back your loans because most of your patients have been trained and conditioned to allow certain insurance companies to choose the healthcare services which they can utilize. You will learn in a short period of time that the insurance companies do not like the principles which you have learned in chiropractic college. These principles are not admired by the petrochemical corporations of the world because they go against the philosophies these companies have taken the time to set up. You have to understand that chiropractic is a drugless healthcare profession (at least it is at the time of this writing) and that the intended objective of chiropractic has traditionally gone against the allopathic model of healthcare that has been engineered by the petrochemical corporations of the world.

Years ago when chiropractic fees were not accepted by insurance companies, our profession existed entirely as a cash business. Patients and doctors, not insurance companies, decided the amount of care that was to be administered. The petrochemical corporations wanted to crush the chiropractic profession in those days because they understood that our profession was slowly becoming stronger each year. Because chiropractic had cash paying patients, it had achieved an unusually large degree of independence which other competing healthcare professions had never enjoyed. Chiropractors and their patients did not have to worry, during this time frame, about answering to third party insurance companies and so there existed a tremendous amount of freedom and growth within the chiropractic industry.

Setting the Trap

The petrochemical corporations of the world decided to set a large trap for the members of the chiropractic profession. Very simply, the goal was to allow insurance plans to begin to cover chiropractic services for the very first time. This strategic maneuver would ultimately allow the petrochemical corporations to gain complete control over the chiropractic profession. The decision to allow chiropractic fees to become eligible for insurance reimbursement immediately opened the doors to the trap and directly invited chiropractors to become dependent on third party insurance companies which were owned by the petrochemical corporations in the first place. When chiropractors agreed to play in the insurance game they swallowed the bait provided by the petrochemical corporations hook, line, and sinker. The leaders of our profession thought that being able to accept insurance was an important victory for chiropractic and that this victory would help to strengthen chiropractic's position in the overall healthcare arena. The chiropractic leaders could not have made a bigger error in their analysis of this scheme.

Once chiropractors were on board it was only a matter of time before the insurance companies of the world began to compensate these doctors for services that were exclusively allopathic in nature. Fees for services that corrected vertebral subluxations were initially paid by the insurance companies with no questions asked. In more recent times it has been an ever increasing amount of therapy fees which have been covered at the highest levels possible while the fees for subluxation correction have been reimbursed minimally or not at all. The total control of the chiropractic profession by the petrochemical corporations of the world has now been completed. If you, as a chiropractor, want to score points in this game that has been designed by these companies you will need to bill for more allopathically based services which the insurance companies will certainly be happy to pay for. You can definitely score some serious points in the contest but in the end you will not be able to win the game because you will have discarded your most valuable assets – your own chiropractic principles.

Getting Out of the Game

If you want to have fun in your practice you will need to get out of the game that has been set up by the petrochemical corporations of the world. Only then will you be able to hang on to your strong principles and only then will you really be free to enjoy what is truly in your heart. Do not make yourself a piece of property that can be owned by a number of greedy corporations. Teach patients the value of your service.

It is possible that in certain situations an insurance product will cover the services you are comfortable providing to your patients and you might be able to coexist with the devil in your practice for limited periods of time. However, if these same insurance companies begin denying your fees because your professional services are not considered important in their eyes, it will be necessary for you to take a stand and to do something about this abuse. In either case you should be teaching your patients to pay for their chiropractic services out of their own pockets. Patients should not rely on insurance plans to pay for their healthcare needs. These plans are all very inadequate and certainly not designed to offer patients ongoing chiropractic wellness care throughout the course of a given year.

If you have the strength and the courage to make these changes within your own office, you are going to be much happier in the long run and you will be able to have a lot more fun in the workplace.

11

Be Persistent

11

Be Persistent

The eleventh secret to becoming a successful chiropractor is to be persistent in whatever it is you are trying to accomplish. It is important to remember that in most situations the effort which you put into a project will have a great deal to do with the type of results which are yielded.

In so many cases the career-related obstacles chiropractors encounter will end up becoming wonderful opportunities for these individuals to experience invaluable professional development. The abilities of certain chiropractors to create direct pathways to success can often be attributed to their constant associations with various professional challenges. Sometimes, the more adversity a professional faces the stronger that person will become.

Earlier in this book, I wrote that a failed attempt by an individual to accomplish a specific objective is actually an opportunity for that person to become successful in accomplishing the same objective at a future date. I believe that this statement really applies to the information I am writing about in this chapter. The professionals in the world who are successful in life are those people who have extraordinary abilities in maintaining the highest levels of determination when situations appear bleak. If you were to take part in a field trip where you could interview many of the successful doctors within the chiropractic profession, I think you would see that many of these practitioners share a similar history in that they did not achieve a high degree of success initially.

Do Not Be Intimidated

Students of chiropractic will often visit successful doctors they know from their home towns who have had established practices for many years. The students observe these highly polished and successful veteran chiropractors in environments which they perceive as being intimidating and then to make matters worse the students will try to compare their own technical skills to that of the professionals which ultimately makes them feel even more inadequate. Students fail to realize that the successful practitioners they are observing have put many hours of dedication and hard work into their profession. These doctors have refined their professional skills as well as their abilities to be successful business people over the course of many long years.

Instant Gratification

One of the biggest threats to a person's ability to become successful is a lack of persistence or determination by the individual who is trying to accomplish a specific goal. Many doctors and students want to achieve every goal which they set for themselves immediately. They want a scenario where immediate results are displayed for whatever it is they are working on. When instant gratification is not attained for a particular objective, these professionals become frustrated and many of them give up on the remainder of their goals.

When you take a look at some of the successes which you have already enjoyed within your own life, you can probably begin to see that most of these accomplishments did not materialize overnight. Most people will observe similar patterns within their own lives and will be able to recognize that goals are attained gradually with little improvements becoming apparent over lengthy periods of time.

Looking back at your career as a student in chiropractic college will help you to put things into a proper perspective. When you started school, you did not earn your degree after the first week of classes. You accomplished getting through school by taking one examination at a time. Do you remember looking through the college's catalogue at all of the courses you were going to have to complete in order to get your degree? It was completely overwhelming to see the unbelievably long list of courses in that college publication. You probably thought that you would never be able to complete such a lengthy program. But you did complete the program and you did earn your degree. Why were you successful in school? The answer is persistence! You were determined to get through each class that you registered for. You were able to break down the bigger experience into smaller objectives and before you realized it you had made it through the entire college program and you received your degree.

Keep Your Goals in Sight

By keeping short and long term goals in sight you will be able to maintain a healthy level of persistence in your own life. On the other hand it will be important for you to be aware of the fact that blind persistence, without any specific objective on your target board, can lead to failure later on.

12

The 33 Chiropractic Principles

12

The 33 Chiropractic Principles

The twelfth secret to becoming a successful chiropractor is being able to fully comprehend the significance of the 33 chiropractic principles. These universal truths are the cornerstones which have offered support and stability to traditional chiropractic since its inception as a healthcare profession. It is quite unfortunate that a rather large number of chiropractors all over the world currently believe that the mere mention of these universal truths make chiropractic look unscientific and more like an organized religion to the rest of the scientific community.

You need to understand that most Americans, as well as other citizens in different countries around the world, have been hypnotized into believing that what they are actually experiencing on a daily basis, is in fact, reality. What you and I are experiencing every day is not a representation of total reality but rather our own limited perception of what we believe reality to be. There is quite a difference between the two concepts.

How Accurate is Science?

According to quantum physicists, there are many different

waves of energy which are present within the third dimensional frequency of existence that we refer to as reality. Unfortunately we do not possess the physical capabilities in our D.N.A. to be able to perceive many of these energy patterns, and so these frequencies are automatically excluded from the equation when we go through the process of forming our own perceptions of reality.

If we, as human beings, do not possess the physical capabilities necessary to be able to view the complete and total reality that makes up the world around us, how can we be so absolutely certain that the scientific research, which many of us cling so desperately to, is in fact accurate when it comes to reporting physical happenings that occur in our world? We have to entertain the possibility that science might not be quite as reliable, when it comes to explaining the physical world, as we might have previously believed.

Trying to Get Outside the Box

As members of society, we are regularly encouraged by others not to make waves and to defend the defined borders of what is commonly known as conventional thinking. Those brave souls who venture "outside the box" of conventional thinking, more often than not, will face a heavy dose of criticism from an unforgiving society which never considers leaving the confinement of such a well-defined safe zone.

Time and time again I have listened to chiropractors try to explain to me that "vertebral subluxations" are not scientifically provable. I have heard these doctors tell me that Straight Chiropractic is based on a religion and that it is not a scientifically-centered healthcare discipline. The arguments that these people present in support of their accusations are based largely on illogical thoughts and many of their assumptions are quite flawed. These folks just hate people who live "outside the box." The claim that a subluxation has never been observed by the human eye is one of the biggest arguments thrown around by doctors who oppose the subluxation practice objective. The skeptics are quick to point out that science needs to unveil the existence of the vertebral subluxation and to make sure that the condition can be made visible for all of the critics to see. Until the vertebral subluxation is made visible by science, these doctors will consider the subluxation practice objective to be nothing more than fantasy.

The same doctors who bash the subluxation practice objective regularly treat headaches, neck pain, low back pain, depression, and a multitude of other conditions that are quite invisible to the human eye. The fact that these doctors cannot visibly see a state of depression in a patient or a headache does not prevent them from treating patients with such conditions. Should doctors stop addressing these problems in patients until science is able to figure out a way to make the conditions visible? I think not.

Chiropractic examination procedures are an accurate and efficient way to measure the damaging effects vertebral subluxations can cause in patients. By measuring certain effects in patients on a regular schedule, we can determine just how detrimental subluxations can be in disrupting the body's physiology.

Is There A Conspiracy?

There are many healthcare practitioners in existence blindly following the allopathic protocols which have been conveniently designed and laid out by the global powers that run the world. It certainly does not take a genius to figure out the reason why allopathy has prospered in the United States and other regions of the world while alternative and more logical approaches to healthcare have struggled. The reason, of course, is due to the billions of dollars that are generated each year by the transnational petrochemical companies which have hijacked the entire healthcare industry. Earlier I wrote about these companies and I discussed how these corporations have hijacked the healthcare industry. Here is the rest of the story.

These companies are owned and operated by some of the wealthiest families on the planet. Known by many scholars in the world as the "Illuminati" these genetically-related bloodlines make up what is secretly known as the "Power Elite." Perhaps you might think this is an attempt by yours truly to create an elaborate conspiracy theory. My suggestion to those individuals falling into this line of reasoning is to invest some personal time to perform a little research about these topics. After you have had the chance to examine some independent news sources which regularly discuss these controversial subjects because they are not contractually bound to the conventional mainstream media companies owned by the illuminati, you might decide to rethink your position about this subject. The next time you get on the Internet go into *"Google"* and type in the word "Illuminati" and then take a good long look at what comes up on your computer screen.

The History of Chiropractic

Let's examine for a moment the long history of calculated attacks by organized medicine against the chiropractic profession. The profession of chiropractic contains a very beneficial healthcare objective – the location, analysis, and correction of vertebral subluxations. Its founder and developer, D.D. and B.J. Palmer obviously had access to information (ancient esoteric knowledge) that had literally been passed on by the "Illuminati" for many thousands of years. The Palmers took that body of knowledge (information that was probably not supposed to be released to the mainstream population) and gave it a completely refurbished name – chiropractic.

As soon as chiropractic was born (1895), there were immediate attempts by the "Illuminati" to try and discredit its validity as a healthcare profession. The stronghold that allopathic medicine placed on the United States and other countries has made it nearly impossible to market chiropractic and its usefulness to the members of the world community. Organized medicine, which was probably the brainchild of the "Illuminati," made sure that chiropractic would never have an easy time becoming accepted as a healthcare profession within the United States or other locations around the world.

Chiropractic represents a direct threat to the allopathic disease management programs that have been unleashed on humanity throughout the entire world. The personal research I have conducted over many years has led me to the inevitable conclusion that allopathy is a lucrative money-maker, a population control manager, and a religion imposed on the world's population. This research has also made me aware of the fact that allopathy has many other components directly attached to it that are even far more sinister.

Allopathy contains multiple mechanisms directly incorporated into its very core which have been mandated by ruling governments or otherwise imposed on the general public. Mechanisms such as these ultimately assure "organized medicine" a never-ending supply of customers (patients) for generations to come. For example, compulsory vaccination programs which have been disguised as disease prevention campaigns are in reality the catalysts which are necessary to transform a healthy community into one that suffers with chronic ailments and is in constant need of allopathic remedies. Indoctrination of the masses via the large consortium of pharmaceutical companies that are literally writing the textbooks utilized in allopathic teaching universities, has created misunderstanding and confusion about health and physiology within the various nations that make up the world community.

It is interesting to note that many forms of "secret knowledge" have been passed on through the eons of time by members of the "Illuminati" so that other members within the same genetic bloodlines could have access to important universal truths. The "secret knowledge" is powerful information about how the laws of the universe really operate. Those individuals with access to such information have quite an advantage over the members of society not having a direct connection to such important information. Much of this knowledge has probably been passed on over many thousands of years by secret societies that have distant but direct connections to the "Mystery Schools" of ancient cultures.

Secret societies come in all shapes and forms. On the surface they may appear very benign or innocuous-looking to members. The secret organizations will usually have 33 levels or degrees of membership and each time a person is promoted to a higher degree within the structure of a secret society, a small ceremony is performed to celebrate the accomplishment of the individual being elevated in status. Each level that members climb in the chapter's order exposes a little more of the "secret knowledge" to them. Much of the information at various lower degrees is inaccurate and purposely given out to confuse initiates. Very few members at the lower end of the spectrum ever advance to levels where they find out the complete truth about the "secret knowledge." Only those individuals with direct genetic connections to the "Illuminati" families from ancient cultures will advance up the organizational ladder within these secret clubs.

Secret societies can be found in college universities, local communities within various countries, and many are built within the framework of religious institutions. The names for these secret organizations can be and usually are different from one another however, underneath these camouflaged titles are powerful networks that are devoted to passing on vital ancient esoteric knowledge to the newer bloodline members which exist on present day Earth.

The Significance of 33

The personal research I have been involved with over the last ten years has allowed me to view certain events that are taking place in the present from a different vantage point than most people and therefore it is quite easy for me to see the hallmark signs that chiropractic has been passed on through the ages under different titles. Perhaps the best tell-tale sign that chiropractic is the direct product of ancient esoteric knowledge is the fact that it is based on "33" written philosophical principles. The number "33" is quite significant because it is the key number which marks the levels of membership in virtually all of the major secret societies that are in existence.

Whenever a universal truth, such as chiropractic, accidentally slips into the public domain it is almost always attacked by the "Illuminati" and made to look unscientific in the eyes of the mainstream scientific community. Whether the citizens of the world realize it or not, mainstream science was bought off long ago by those people in the know who wanted to keep humanity firmly positioned within that small box known as "conventionality." The ancient esoteric knowledge that has been passed on through the ages by the "Illuminati" has been carefully hidden from the general population. It is intentionally kept out of mainstream circulation.

Are We Witnessing the Death of a Profession?

Today doctors of chiropractic are witnessing the death of a wonderful profession. Chiropractic and its principles have been under attack for quite a long time. In recent years, the allopathic monopolized healthcare system has captured the key organizations which regulate and evaluate the professional standards within the chiropractic profession. As has been the case in the past with other alternative healthcare professions that have stepped "out of the box" such as osteopathy and naturopathy, chiropractic is currently in the final stages of being absorbed by modern medicine so that it can be redesigned with a brand new practice objective.

Chiropractors in the future will have to support allopathic protocols and will have to endorse vaccination programs as well as many other components of the medical agenda. If things continue to move along at the current pace, the chiropractic profession along with its objective of correcting vertebral subluxations will disappear within a few more years. If doctors of chiropractic do not take aggressive actions soon to stop the damage being done by allopathy and the chiropractic organizations that are secretly working for "organized medicine" while posing disingenuously as institutions trying to advance chiropractic, then we chiropractors along with our profession will become just another casualty of allopathic protocol!

As a doctor of chiropractic you need to understand that the 33 chiropractic principles which our profession is based upon are solid universal truths. The chiropractic principles are essential to the continued existence of our profession. These principles have stood up to the test of time and they have endured the attacks of many well-organized groups. The principles are as valid today as they were one hundred years ago and they will be just as valid one hundred years from now into the future.

Universal truths do not need to be modified because they are inherently perfect. By following these practice principles you will be taking a major step in ensuring your own eventual success as a doctor of chiropractic.

13

Support the Major Disciplines Within Your Profession Equally

13

Support the Major Disciplines Within Your Profession Equally

The thirteenth secret to becoming a successful chiropractor is to learn how to support the major disciplines within your profession equally. If chiropractic is to survive well into the future, it will be necessary for its practitioners to understand the importance of these disciplines as vital components within the chiropractic profession.

Traditionally-based chiropractic has acquired much of its strength from three major disciplines known as _art_, _science_, and _philosophy_. Chiropractic shares a unique relationship with these disciplines and over the years many chiropractic scholars have discussed in detail the importance of maintaining balance between art, science, and philosophy. If the chiropractic profession is to remain strong, it will need to maintain this delicate balance in the years to come.

Art

The artistic aspect of chiropractic deals specifically with various technical components which are important to the overall success of the profession. The analyses and corrective procedures which regularly allow chiropractors options in maintaining proper spinal integrity for patients are merely different forms of artistic expression.

Chiropractic students often become obsessed with studying certain techniques. They incorrectly believe, at various stages of their education, that a particular technique package is superior to other analytical and corrective procedures. This is a very natural process that students have to work through and it is quite normal for future chiropractors to become overly excited about certain techniques which they are learning in the classroom. This is especially true when students are studying corrective procedures for the very first time. I have always encouraged my students to learn as many techniques as possible. Information that does not sit well with an individual can always be discarded at a later date.

The more seasoned chiropractor will understand that techniques are merely tools utilized to complete a particular professional objective. The value of any given technique is measured by its ability or lack of ability to accomplish the profession's intended objective. I personally have never been married to a specific technique. Instead, I have always utilized a collection of tools which allowed me the opportunity to complete my professional objective of locating, analyzing, and correcting vertebral subluxations in my patients.

Depending on the scenario and other contributing factors that can play into the equation, one technique might work more efficiently than another corrective procedure for a specific patient. This does not mean, by any stretch of the imagination, that this particular technique is superior to other tools in the shed.

The artistic aspect of chiropractic, although extremely important, would be quite meaningless and very insignificant without the presence of philosophy and science. A collection of tools is quite impractical if you do not have a rationale or objective in mind for their use. You could have the most elaborate analytical and corrective procedures in existence but without a specific professional objective to set your sights on, the procedures would be absolutely pointless.

Science

When introduced into a relationship with chiropractic, science can be described as a branch of knowledge that helps us to explain the physical and biological properties which routinely occur in human beings. The first cousin of science, which is known as research, can also be helpful in documenting statistical data that is imperative for measuring progress in accomplishing goals as well as measuring the effectiveness or ineffectiveness of certain forms of artistic expression being routinely utilized by practitioners on patients.

Science, as it relates to chiropractic, is often over-emphasized by some of the members within our profession and this can be very detrimental to the important balance that exists between these three disciplines of knowledge. The collection of statistical data which culminates in the stockpiling of mounds of information that explain biological and physical properties is rather useless unless you have technical components which can utilize the pertinent materials being collected.

Philosophy

Philosophy is also an integral part of the chiropractic profession. Without a professional rationale, which regularly encourages us to accomplish various goals, we would most likely not have a functioning profession. Philosophy which explains the "why" of everything that is chiropractic provides a course of direction for the proper utilization of science and its related fields.

As important as philosophy is to chiropractic it still must be supported at all times by the disciplines of art and science in order for it to have any meaningful impact on the lives of patients and practitioners. It would be completely illogical to have a philosophical rationale in place for an entire profession while simultaneously excluding artistic and scientific components that would create and validate pathways for the realization of such worthy objectives.

If we take a moment to look back through our turbulent history, we should be able to recognize that our greatest strength as a profession has always been our ability to maintain a healthy balance between art, science, and philosophy. We need to encourage the members of our profession to continue to support all three of these important disciplines equally. Keeping the three disciplines on a level playing field will ensure all chiropractors opportunities to have successful professional careers.

14

Keep Informed
About Your Profession

14

Keep Informed
About Your Profession

The fourteenth secret to becoming a successful chiropractor is to keep informed about your profession. There are many industry related events that professionals must pay attention to on a regular basis. Doctors will need to have a reliable way to monitor various developments that might directly or indirectly affect the chiropractic profession as well as their professional practices.

So many chiropractors have apathetic attitudes about the political happenings taking place within the profession. I believe that many practitioners are lulled into a false sense of security when it comes to internal affairs such as these. A genuine lack of desire by a majority of the members residing within the chiropractic profession to get involved with various political organizations has paved the way for many of the detrimental changes that have recently occurred within the framework of the chiropractic profession.

I understand that it is often difficult for private practitioners to clear enough time from their busy schedules so that they can attend meetings which are being held at distant locations. While it might not be practical for doctors to physically attend every meeting or event scheduled within an organization's calendar, it certainly is possible for most doctors to join and support the key organizations that are supporting and fighting for their rights to practice a specific professional objective.

Chiropractors can become involved with professional organizations that are important to the continued survival of the profession without giving up a lot of their precious time. By joining professional coalitions and paying membership fees, chiropractors can help support these organizations. In addition to monies which are collected from club members, many of these organizations gain or lose power and political clout just from the number of doctors that are officially registered with a specific organization.

Chiropractors who are registered members of such organizations can receive newsletters and transcripts from official meetings which they are unable to attend. A doctor need not attend every meeting to become aware of the important issues that are regularly being addressed.

I have previously discussed in this book the challenges that chiropractors often face when dealing with time management issues. The doctors who decide to join professional chiropractic organizations, which have the resources to keep their members informed of important political and legislative happenings, are to be commended for managing their own time very effectively. These doctors are, in a sense, delegating the work of keeping themselves updated about important professional issues to specialized organizations and at the same time are able to manage their own time very efficiently. The doctors who are members of these organizations are able to stay informed of various political happenings that are very important to the entire chiropractic profession. This becomes a winning situation for everyone concerned and it helps to get large numbers of chiropractors to take an interest in important professional issues.

I Practice What I Preach

I honestly believe that every chiropractor should make it a point to join a professional organization that represents his or her practice rationale. I am currently a member of the Federation of Straight Chiropractors and Organizations. I support this organization and encourage others within the profession that I come into contact with to do the same. I do not have the resources or the time to keep abreast of every important issue that faces our great profession; however I do feel comfortable and confident in writing that this organization is working diligently to keep me informed about pertinent information that is vital to my own continued success.

Because I believe that it is extremely important to learn as much as possible about what is going on in the chiropractic profession, I will continue to be a member of the FSCO and I will continue to rely heavily on this organization to keep me informed about important professional issues. It is my friendly advice to all chiropractors to try and do the same.

15

Think like a Business Person

15

Think like a Business Person

The fifteenth and final secret to becoming a successful chiropractor is to be able to think like a business person when operating your practice. A small percentage of the doctors in our profession are gifted business people and they have very few problems if any when it comes to managing their professional practices. Other doctors however, will struggle quite a bit with business-related obstacles and they never do seem to get their offices up and running properly.

Many chiropractors just starting out have little or no experience in operating a business. The nuts and bolts of running a practice are not always thoroughly covered in every chiropractic college. Some schools will offer courses that cover basic business strategies, however many students are not focused on these issues when they are navigating their way through classes. Most students are primarily concerned with learning how to become competent doctors and how to get through the four sections of the National Board. So even though business subjects are sometimes presented in college courses, many students are unable to absorb this vital information.

Regardless of whether or not an individual is equipped with the proper skills to succeed in a particular practice setting it is important to realize that certain business skills are necessary to make a practice run properly. If you do not know what you are doing in the business world you could very easily find yourself in a lot of trouble within a very short period of time. Some chiropractors manage to get into serious trouble in just a few months.

There are many items that must be dealt with when setting up or running a chiropractic business. A few of these business challenges are listed below:

*Financial Strategies
*Insurance Concerns
*Negotiating Leases
*Advertising Campaigns
*Equipment Concerns
*Tax Preparation Procedures
*Patient Management Procedures
*Patient Education Procedures
*Paperwork Concerns
*Borrowing Money

Obviously, I am only scratching the surface with the items that I have placed on this list. The point that I am trying to make is that when it comes right down to it you have to be able to make good business decisions on a regular basis so that your practice has the best chance to survive in an environment that is sometimes very non forgiving.

Keep Your Overhead Low

One of the most important things that you can do to ensure your own success as a business person is to try and keep your expenses (office overhead) low. Every dollar that you spend in the daily operation of your office must be earned back in the form of business income. While it is true that you have to spend money to make money, you should also be aware of the fact that spending company money foolishly can lead to bigger problems in the future.

Chiropractors routinely spend a lot more money than they have to when it comes to setting up a functional office. Sometimes you have to think like a business person and not like a chiropractor. You have to evaluate what types of equipment, office space, furniture, supplies, and other items are necessary for the smooth operation of your facility. Is it really necessary to spend fifteen thousand dollars for a brand new adjusting table? Could you adequately take care of patients on a refurbished table that only costs eight hundred dollars? Learn to make good business decisions by evaluating situations based on facts and not your emotions.

Educate Yourself

If you lack the business skills that I have been writing about in this chapter, you will need to take a trip to your local library so that you can check out some books that discuss basic business procedures. I also highly recommend that you pick up a copy of the book that I co-authored in 2002 entitled *"Up and Running: Opening a Chiropractic Office"* PageFree Publishing, Inc. ISBN 1930252706. This book will, in very simple terms, show you how to avoid the pitfalls of costly practice mistakes as well as how to get your chiropractic office up and running in an affordable and professional manner.

Remember that your office is a business and if you want to keep it around for a long time you will need to run it properly. Learn to think like a business person and you will be well on your way to having a long and successful career as a chiropractor.

Afterword

You now know the fifteen secrets to becoming a successful chiropractor. If you make an honest effort to follow the formula which I have outlined in this book, I believe that you will be able to embrace a tremendous amount of success in the very near future.

I want to reiterate once again that just knowing about a set of secrets is not going to be enough to get the job done. You will need to take action and you will need to start doing the things that I have been writing about immediately. Do not wait for tomorrow to start your plan of action. Take an aggressive approach and begin implementing your own strategies for success right away.

You will most likely have to read the fifteen secrets several times in order to get the maximum benefit out of the material. Never give up trying to accomplish the goals that you have set for yourself. In addition, try to remember that it takes a lot of hard work and dedication to be able to accomplish a specific goal.

I hope that you have enjoyed reading this book and I hope that I have made you aware of the unlimited potential for success which you already possess.

- Dr. John Reizer

Printed in the United States
97120LV00004B/5/A

9 781589 613607